GW00374912

Heidi Grollmann, Urs Maurer
Understanding Classical Homœopathy

Heidi Grollmann, Urs Maurer

Understanding
Classical Homœopathy

The foundations of Classical Homœopathy

English translation by Hans G. Schrauder

Groma Verlag Baar

© Copyright Groma Verlag
Oberdorfstrasse 2, 6340 Baar, Switzerland
www.groma.ch, E-Mail: groma@groma.ch
All rights reserved

German Title: Klassische Homöopathie verstehen
1. Edition January 1996
2. Edition July 1996
3. Edition September 1997
4. Edition January 2001
5. Edition May 2002

English translation by Hans G. Schrauder
1. Edition July 2002

A catalogue record for this book is available from the British Library

Sales and distribution enquiries to:

Hans G. Schrauder, Interlink Systems Ltd, 82 Amberwood Rise, New Malden, Surrey KT3 5JQ, United Kingdom
Email: the.homoeopath@virgin.net

ISBN 3-9521004-2-0

Content

Preface

1st – 3rd Edition

We noticed, in our daily work with our patients, that there was a great need for an easily understandable introduction to Classical Homœopathy.

We were particularly requested to explain the basis of Classical Homœopathy, since it is so often confused with other alternative health practices. It is, in fact, an independent science with its own laws. Furthermore, a well-informed patient can better understand the course of his or her treatment contributing to a speedier recovery.

These methods of treatment require a different understanding of health and disease. The patient must be prepared to confront his illness and the healing process.

With this book, and a variety of seminars, we wish to add to the amount of information available and to bring Classical Homœopathy to a wider audience.

4th Edition

The large demand – over 10 000 copies sold in German-speaking Europe – and the many positive comments from colleagues and patients have given us great pleasure. This shows, that Classical Homœopathy is well established and widespread.

Now we have the fourth corrected edition ready. We reviewed and expanded the entire content. The following innovations enhance this edition: we supplemented the various chapters with case histories taken from everyday practice. The chapter on the Miasms has been greatly expanded after many requests from various quarters. The chapter on Constitutional Treatment is new, as is the chapter on Frequently Asked Questions in daily practice.

At this point, we wish to thank all those who helped to add to this new edition with their various comments. Also our thanks to Brigitte Kurath and Kathrin Büchi-Möller for their invaluable support.

Heidi Grollmann   Urs Maurer

Translator's Foreword

This book will always remind me of the beautiful Greek island of Alonissos. I first came to know of the book during an International Open Teaching Seminar on Homœopathy, taught by George Vithoulkas, on Alonissos. It is such a beautifully produced and simple text, and I just knew that the English-speaking world would want to have the benefit of its easy and attractive introduction to Classical Homœopathy.

Patients and future patients of homœopathy will find in this book a clear and easily understandable introduction to the basics of the most powerful system of medicine in the world.

This book will appeal to all homœopaths who have been looking for a simple text that communicates to their patients the essence of what we, as homoeopaths, do and why we ask such an awful lot of strange questions. I expect it to be on sale in most homœopathic practices that wish their patients to be as informed as possible about the nature of their treatment.

The authors of this book, Heidi Grollmann and Urs Maurer, are two of the nicest people and most passionate homœopaths that I have ever had the privilege of meeting. They run a busy practice, a thriving School for Classical Homœopathy, seminars for professional and lay-person alike, write very appealing books on homœopathy, and still find time to run marathons and holes into the Zurich pavements.

All the wisdom and creativity is theirs, all the faults mine.

Hans G. Schrauder BSc LCH MHMA MGCP

Samuel Hahnemann (1755–1843)

Founder of Homœopathy

Christian Friedrich Samuel Hahnemann, the founder and discoverer of homœopathy, was born in Meissen on the 12th of April 1755, the son of a porcelain painter. Financial circumstances were anything but rosy at that time. Because of his exceptional talent, he nonetheless found a patron that enabled him to go to High School. In order to study medicine in Leipzig, he was obliged to pay his way by giving foreign-language tuition and performing translation work. He was one of the most respected translators of his time. By the age of 24 he commanded seven languages both written and spoken. In 1779 he sat his doctorate examinations in Erlangen.

Shortly after commencing practice he became disillusioned about medicine. Excessive bloodletting, brutal vomiting and laxative cures often ended fatally. Powerful medication made from Lead, Mercury or Arsenic poisoned the patients. Hahnemann protested loudly against these damaging and ineffective methods that were then normal. Soon, his colleagues were accusing him of heresy. Hahnemann gave up his practice in disappointment. He supported himself by translating medical works.

During the translation of a pharmacopoeia by Dr Cullen (1790), he was troubled by the explanation for the action of China bark on malaria, namely that it was due to its astringent effects on the stomach. This assertion struck him as unlikely. He decided on a self-experiment and took the China bark himself. He resolved to test its effects on the healthy organism, and repeatedly took this herbal remedy until his body reacted with a fever, shivering, and various other symptoms of malaria.

From this Hahnemann concluded that malaria was cured by China bark, not because of its astringent action on the stomach, but by the fact that this medicine produces the symptoms of malaria in the healthy.

For six years, following this groundbreaking discovery, Hahnemann carried out experiments on himself and family members, using various substances. Increasingly, Hahnemann turned again to the practice of medicine. He did not shy away from questioning generally accepted truths and sought his own explanations. Thus, he represented a serious threat to established medicine.

Hahnemann coined the expression "homœopathy". This came from the Greek "homoios" (similar) and "pathos" (suffering). He recommended the use of only single remedies, which, in addition, he prescribed in small doses. Because of this, dispensing chemists became his greatest enemies, since they feared for their businesses. Despite continual persecution, homœopathy continued to develop.

His major work "The Organon of the Art of Healing" appeared in 1810. The basic laws and principles of homœopathy, which remain valid to the present time, are recorded therein. The multiple volume work "The Chronic Diseases" appeared between 1828–1830.

In 1835, the widowed Hahnemann married a young Frenchwoman. He moved with his new wife to Paris. This last episode in Hahnemann's life was very important for the expansion of homœopathy. For eight years, Hahnemann ran an extensive practice in Paris. He led it successfully until just a few weeks before his death. Hahnemann died at the age of 88, on the 2nd of July 1843. He lies buried in "Père Lachaise", the cemetery for the distinguished in Paris. His grave with its impressive tombstone can still be visited.

The Law of Similars

Similia similibus curentur

The basis of homœopathy is the "law of similars". "Similia similibus curentur". "Similars are to be healed with similars", i. e., an illness can only be healed with that homœopathic remedy, which produces similar symptoms in a healthy person.

What should be understood by that? You have a cold, complain of tears in your eyes, itching or burning eyes, tickling in the nose, attacks of sneezing and have developed a watery, acrid, sore producing nasal secretion. Only the homœopathic remedy that is capable of producing these symptoms in someone healthy can help you.

This symptom picture occurs when you are cutting onions. Within a short while the above-mentioned symptoms of burning eyes, acrid nasal secretions etc. appear. Should you now develop the same or similar symptoms as with the previously mentioned cold, the remedy Allium cepa, made from the common onion, would cure this cold.

To clarify the Law of Similars, a second example: you certainly recognise the condition of excess consumption of coffee. Depending on individual sensitivity, many people develop complaints such as nervousness, shaking, palpitations, sleeplessness etc. The homœopathic remedy Coffea (coffee) would often be prescribed for the above-mentioned symptoms.

That like can heal like is already mentioned in the ancient writings of the Greek doctor Hippocrates (460 to 377 BC). Paracelsus (1493 to 1541) hinted at this principle in his works.

However, Hahnemann was the first to pursue this knowledge with thoroughness and persistence and develop it into a well-founded method of healing.

Disease and Cure

A question of the Vital Force

efore we occupy ourselves with the cure, we must settle exactly what disease actually is.

- Why does one catch the flu while the other remains healthy, although both came in contact with the same flu patient?

- Why does one person react to the enjoyment of food with massive skin eruptions while the other can eat it unscathed?

- Why can a good pupil quite calmly sit an exam while the other, equally good, pupil fails the exam from anxiety?

- Why are some people susceptible to something and others not?

Homœopathy intensely addressed these questions and concluded that a superior energy called the Vital Force or Dynamis steers all the functions of life.

The task of the Vital Force is to maintain harmony and order in the organism. Every component of the organism, every organ and every cell is influenced and guarded by the Vital Force. The Vital Force protects us from illness and confers immunity against factors inducing disease.

As soon as the Vital Force is weakened or out of balance, e. g. through strain, stress, mental problems etc., a person becomes ill. The organism is no longer protected from the causes of disease, e. g. bacteria, viruses, fungi, pollen, stress etc. Only a disturbed Vital Force causes disease.

Changes to tissue or organs, e. g. inflammation, ulcers, deformed joints, cysts etc., are not themselves the disease, rather the results of the disease process. They are simply indicating that something is not right inside the person. The patient isn't ill because he has a tumour; rather the tumour is there because the patient is ill.

Indeed, viruses and bacteria are never the true cause of disease. It is the weakened Vital Force that encourages the growth of foreign organisms such as bacteria, viruses and fungi. That means, first comes the disturbance of the Vital Force, and then the agent spreads.

When the symptoms of an illness are removed, either surgically, e.g. the removal of haemorrhoids, or through medicinal action, e.g. the treatment of eczema with the use of strong acting ointments, then that doesn't mean by a long shot that the illness is conquered.

The origins of the illness are to be found in the weakened Vital Force. Medication or an operation solely deals with the end result of the disease process. The disturbance of the Vital Force is not removed with these treatments. The illness can spread itself further and cause new damage to other parts of the organism.

It follows therefore that true cure is only possible through harmonising the Vital Force.

Homœopathic remedies influence the Vital Force, stimulate the self-healing forces of the sick person, return him to equilibrium and thus strengthen the Vital Force. The person is supported in healing himself.

Individuality

Everyone is different

A very important rule in Classical Homœopathy is the view that every person is unique. The individual observation of the patient is the most important fundamental task of the homœopath. It is always the single, unmistakable person that is being treated. He becomes ill in his own particular way and produces his own symptoms. Thus, the appropriate remedy for him must be found that no other can replace. Hence, it is less important for the homœopath what disease or diagnosis the patient has, rather how the particular illness manifests itself in the patient.

Let us take as an illustration, the widespread complaint "headache".

- *One patient had a point of pain over the root of the nose.*
- *A second complains of pulsating pains in the forehead.*
- *Another has dull pains at the back of the head.*

The circumstances under which the complaint is made better or worse play an important role.

- *One patient with headache feels better with warmth.*
- *Another better with cold compresses and when he presses his fingers on the painful spot.*
- *With the third, the complaint is relieved by lying down in the dark and worsened by glaring light.*

The cause of an illness must also be thoroughly studied.

- *One patient was caught in a thunderstorm while out walking. He thus caught a cold and as a result developed a sinusitis with a strong headache.*

- *Another was in the sun too long and now suffers from resulting sunstroke.*

Psychological triggers are to be taken into account. Worries, grief, financial loss, jealousy, stress etc., can all cause illness.

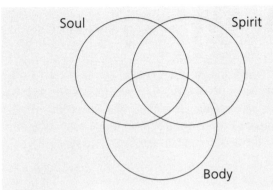

Homœopathy views people as a unity of body, mind and spirit. It is not possible to separate these. Because of this, the character and mood of the patient plays a very important role. The one is introverted, has everything under control, suppresses his emotions, appears unapproachable, and blocked. Another is moody, aggressive, and impulsive with no signs of reserve or love of fellow human beings. He is best avoided.

Previous health disturbances, illnesses in the family and other details also give valuable pointers to finding the remedy (see Chapters: *The Miasmatic Disposition & Case Taking in the Practice).*

The Classical Homœopath, with the assistance of an individual's symptoms, searches for a remedy that is attuned to the patient. The appropriate medicine for each patient will be sought drawing on knowledge and a capacity to empathise.

The homœopath does not prescribe a remedy that has the name of the disease (e. g., headache) written on it, rather seeks a remedy that meets the total state of the patient. So 10 patients, all suffering the same condition (e. g. headaches) could receive 10 different medicines each according to their individual symptoms.

Homœopathy – Allopathy

Totally different philosophies

Homœopathy and allopathy (orthodox medicine) have a quite different understanding of health and disease as their basis. In the previous chapter, we explained these issues from a homœopathic viewpoint. As already mentioned, in homœopathy, sickness is equated to a disturbance in the Vital Force, health with a return to harmony of the Vital Force.

In orthodox medicine, on the other hand, the symptoms are seen as the disease itself. When, for example, a growth is operated on, the patient is subsequently regarded as healthy. Should new complaints occur in other organs after the operation, these will be viewed as manifestations of a new illness and nobody will give any thought to a possible connection to the operation.

A skin eruption that disappears after the application of an ointment is regarded as cured. In allopathy, an illness must be measurable, visible, detectable with the aid of the laboratory, microscope, X-ray, ultrasound, CT scanner etc. As soon as values are normal and signs of sickness have disappeared, the patient is viewed as cured. The true condition of the patient is of lesser importance, since it cannot be measured or be made objectively visible.

In homœopathy, however, these visible signs of disease are all only the result of an internal disturbance and illness. The real illness is deeper, namely in the disturbance of the Vital Force, and is thus invisible.

In allopathic thinking, bacteria, viruses, fungi and other microbes are the cause of illness and must be radically killed off with antibiotics and fungicides.

Homœopaths, on the other hand, have the view that foreign germs can only lodge themselves and cause damage in a weakened organism. The defences of the organism must be strengthened, and then to a great extent, people would be spared disease. Homœopathy does not kill bacteria or fungi, rather strengthens the person so that he is no longer susceptible to disease.

Homœopathy is not against life preserving operations or against accident and emergency medicine, which can give valuable service, especially with injuries and assisting in labour and childbirth. A broken bone cannot be healed homœopathically, it must be set and put in plaster. But one can accelerate the healing process with homœopathy.

Also, within health care there are purely mechanical problems, especially in chronic illness, e.g. growths that, when widespread, can affect or even prevent the functioning of organs. Hence we cannot possibly do without surgery, especially where mechanical blockages make an operation necessary.

Surgery, however, doesn't cure disease; rather it removes the result of an illness, which could possibly have been prevented if one had commenced homœopathic treatment in time.

In recent decades, various operations have repeatedly crossed the country, like a fashion statement. For years all children had their tonsils removed, whether they had persistent sore throats or not. Only a few decades ago in Switzerland, certain professions were required to have their tonsils removed (for safety reasons!) before taking up their post. In this way one wanted to prevent a civil servant from getting a sore throat and possibly infecting other colleagues.

Not only tonsils but also other organs were and still are removed unnecessarily, for example, the womb. In the Federal Republic of Germany today, every third woman over the age of 40 no longer has a womb. With postmenopausal women the figure rises to 53 percent, and in Switzerland, according to the Zurich Cancer Register of 1994, one third of all 50 to 70 year-old women are affected.

In allopathy, each patient with a particular complaint receives a similar medication, for example, with pain – a pain-killer, with rheumatism – a rheumatism medicine, with hay-fever – an antihistamine, with skin eruptions – cortisone etc.

In homœopathy, a remedy will be prescribed according to the individual symptoms of the patient (see Chapter: *Individuality*).

Homœopathy views people as a single entity, an inseparable whole of body, mind, and spirit. It is always the entirety that is treated, not just the separate pieces.

In allopathy, there is ever more specialisation. A heart case is referred to a cardiologist, with gastrointestinal disturbances an internal medicine specialist leaps into action. Research progresses more and more and thus ever more specialist fiefdoms develop. But with this search for the singular there is the danger that the person in his entirety is forgotten.

The goal of homœopathic treatment is not to directly remove or suppress a symptom, rather to strengthen and harmonise the Vital Force. The organism is thus placed in a position where it can conquer the disease itself.

In allopathy, one wants to remove the symptoms as quickly as possible, then the patient passes for cured.

In homœopathy, one gives the organism time to become healthy.

As you will clearly see, the basic tenants of both these therapies are totally different. Because of this, homœopathy is often attacked and its successes disputed, since its laws cannot be understood or researched from the point of view of orthodox medicine.

Homœopathic Medicines

Preparation and potentising

Sources

Homœopathic medicines are made from the following substances:

- **Plants, e. g.** Club Moss (Lycopodium), Deadly Nightshade (Belladonna), Wind-flower (Pulsatilla).

- **Animals, e. g.** Bees (Apis), Ants (Formica rufa), snake poisons e. g., Bushmaster Snake (Lachesis).

- **Metals, e. g.** Copper (Cuprum metallicum), Gold (Aurum metallicum), Iron (Ferrum metallicum).

- **Minerals, e. g.** Carbonate of lime/Chalk (Calcium carbonicum), Flint (Silicea), Phosphate of magnesia (Magnesium phosphoricum).

- **Products of disease,** so-called Nosodes.

- **Acids, e. g.** Nitric acid (Nitricum acidum), Phosphoric acid (Phosphoricum acidum).

- and others.

Preparation

Homœopathic drugs are prepared by a special process. Soluble materials are diluted and shaken (succussed) in stages, insoluble substances such as Gold, Iron, Quartz, etc. are dissolved step-by-step and ground up in milk sugar (Lactose).

This dilution in stages is called Potentising (energising). The healing power of many substances is only released, and the toxicity of poisonous substances is only lost by potentisation. This explains for example, that un-potentised Petroleum is completely useless as a remedy. Potentised however, it realises its curative action and becomes a valuable medicine, e. g. for travel sickness, skin problems, or headaches, as long as it is prescribed according to a patient's individual requirements.

Potency

There are various potencies. Most useful are the so-called C-potencies (Centesimal potencies). These are prepared as follows:

One part starting substance is dissolved in 99 parts alcohol/water mixture and shaken. This gives the potency 1C. From this 1C, again one part is dissolved in 99 parts alcohol/water mixture and shaken; giving us a 2C, etc.

If the dissolving is done in steps off 10, namely one part of starting material is dissolved in nine parts of alcohol/water mixture and shaken, then one speaks of X-potencies or D-potencies (decimal potencies). These are used largely in Germany.

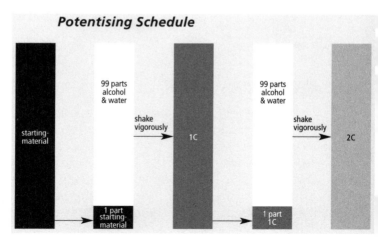

Potentising Schedule

starting-material

99 parts alcohol & water

shake vigorously

1 part starting-material

1C

99 parts alcohol & water

shake vigorously

1 part 1C

2C

The precise preparation processes for each remedy are described in the homœopathic pharmacopoeia. Apart from the C- and X-potencies, Q- or LM-potencies have established themselves. These consist of dilution steps of 1:50 000.

Effectiveness

Potentised medicines from 12C or 23X onwards no longer have a single molecule left. It is merely the information of the remedy that is transferred to the alcohol/water mixture or milk sugar. This information is not [currently] detectable in the laboratory. Chemically, only the carrier substance can be analysed. Thus, science asserts that homœopathic remedies above 23X cannot have any effect since they no longer contain a single molecule of starting material.

For a better understanding of the effectiveness of homœopathic remedies, here are two examples:

> You are holding our book in your hand and are reading these lines at this moment. We have put our thoughts to paper. This paper, upon which we have written the information, is the information carrier. If this book were to be chemically analysed, one would have examined merely the information carrier and broken it into its constituent parts. But in this analysis the most important thing would be lost, namely the information that was on the paper. That cannot be identified by any method.

> Or take a video or music cassette and weigh it. Now record on the cassette and weigh it anew. You will establish that the weight of the recorded cassette is the same as the weight of the unrecorded, although information has been saved on it.

Naturally, this is only an attempt at an explanation, and like every hypothesis is not 100 percent applicable. In many areas of life there are phenomena that cannot be scientifically explained. This does not mean that they do not exist.

Homœopathic remedies are non-material, dynamised remedies. As we have already suggested, disease is a dynamic disturbance of the organism. This can only be brought back into balance with dynamic remedies. Homœopathic medicine influences the weakened Vital Force, releasing the healing process.

That homœopathic remedies are effective is undeniable. Indeed, some time ago a study by Scottish researchers at Glasgow University was published in the scientific medical journal "The Lancet", clearly proving this on the basis of patient studies. Even opponents of homœopathy could not refute this study.

Further scientific studies can be found on our website *www.groma.ch*

The Remedy Proving

Testing drugs the safe way –
no animals involved!

The so-called "proving" is an important tenant of homœopathy. It is very demanding and conducted according to special rules. The proving serves to establish the exact effect of a homœopathic substance, i.e. it is a testing process that shows which symptoms a medication can produce and thus also heal.

In a remedy proving, a group of healthy people of both sexes take the substance to be tested in accordance with the regulations. Naturally, these people do not know which substance is involved. Every subsequent change in how they feel is written down and protocolled.

All differences in bodily or mental state are important. Sensations have to be accurately recorded. For example:

- Indifference to his family

- Dreams of amusing things

- Aching back pain radiating to the left leg, which is better for cold and movement

- Stabbing pains in the left knee as if with needles

- etc.

At the end of the proving, the observations are collected together and evaluated and the results form the so-called remedy picture. The remedy picture is added to by clinical observations, which are the experiences from using that remedy on the sick.

The results of all this research are collated together in a homœopathic Materia Medica. It is the most comprehensive collection of remedies that we know.

Animal research in provings is useless since animals cannot describe their sensations or moods. Furthermore, they do not react in the same way as humans. So there is no need for torturous animal experimentation in order to draw conclusions on the effectiveness of medicines. Instead, a healthy person makes himself or herself available for the remedy proving, as described above.

Homœopathic
Remedy Dosage

Using homœopathic remedies

The patient is often astonished when he gets only a few globules or "poppy seeds" that he is to take the next morning on an empty stomach. He asks whether that can be enough, his next appointment is, after all, weeks or even months away.

In Classical Homœopathy, dosages are kept to a minimum. A single push is enough to influence the Vital Force. Repeat the remedy too early and too often and the harmonic healing process will be disturbed. One must give the remedy time to react. Too often a repetition unsettles the Vital Force and brings further disharmony.

To clarify, let us look at a pendulum clock. The clock has stopped. We pull the weight up, give the pendulum a light push and it swings rhythmically to and fro. Touch the pendulum again after a short while, and it becomes unsettled and a short while later the clock stops. As long as something is moving, it does not require additional energy input, otherwise the whole lot ends up on the wrong tracks.

It is a widely held misconception that a homœopathic remedy can do no damage, no matter what the circumstances are. If someone takes the same homœopathic remedy over a longer period, there exists the danger of an undesired remedy proving, i.e. the patient produces the symptoms of the remedy he is taking for curative purposes.

Recently a young man came to the practice with a diagnosis from his doctor of pneumonia. Before, he had received from a so-called "homœopath", and sadly also taken, the alternating homœopathic remedies Tuberculinum and Luesinum in high potency.

*It was explained to the patient that, although he had th
symptoms of pneumonia these were the results of th
misuse of homœopathic remedies, and he was in th
middle of a remedy proving.*

*One dose of Sulphur 200C (a commonly used remed
with drug misuse) and two days later the complaint wa
gone.*

*It should be pointed out that he had never had lun
problems, other than that one instance of pneumonia*

A further example of an undesired remedy proving

*A 52 year-old patient had complained for months of
migraine-like headache leading to nausea and pain on
the right side of the face, with pain radiating into th
right eye. When lifting her arm, or lying upon it at night
she noticed strong pains in her right upper arm and
shoulder joints. Rheumatological and neurological ex
aminations revealed nothing. As an aside, she men
tioned that she had been given a homœopathic remed
by her gynaecologist for menopause complaints that sh
had been taking for a good two years (15 drops two
times daily).*

*Now what had the one to do with the other? The meno
pause drops contained, among other things, the ho
mœopathic remedy Sanguinaria. This remedy has in it
remedy picture a migraine-like right sided headache
right side shoulder pains worse for lying on and when
attempting to lift the arm.*

*Through the excessive consumption of the "menopause
complaint remedy" an undesired remedy proving had
taken place. After stopping the complex remedy and
taking a dose of Nux vomica 200C, the patient was free
from discomfort in a week.*

The higher the potency, the deeper and longer lasting the effect, and the less frequent the remedy should be repeated. High potency remedies have a depot affect. They work for months. Mostly, they are dispensed as globules. In acute illness, it is sometimes sensible to dissolve them in water and drink in sips. Your homœopath will advise you about this. The L.M. potencies are mostly dispensed as drops. They are, as a rule, taken more often than the C and X potencies.

Lower potencies are dispensed in very deep health disturbances, with a severely weakened Vital Force, since a remedy reaction could overburden the organism.

"Single" vs. "Complex" Remedies

The true art of the homœopath lies in finding the correct homœopathic remedy. For that, much knowledge, time, patience and experience is required. One cannot practice homœopathy "on the side", and from a true Classical viewpoint, a working homœopath would not utilise any other form of therapy.

Other forms of therapy and methods

In recent years, the expression "homœopathy" has far too often been used (or abused) for different forms of therapy. Before, one used to say, "I am going to a naturopath" today it is "I am going to a homœopath".

When a therapist looks into our eyes, in other words uses Iridology, and from this can see all our complaints and predispositions, prescribes Phytotherapies, Spagyric Essences or Bach Flower Remedies, then this has nothing to do with Classical Homœopathy, rather these are other distinct modes of healing.

Other therapists want to shorten the demanding route to finding the correct remedy. There has always been a tendency to simplify homœopathy to make it easier to market. For a few years, it has now been fashionable to test for the correct remedy using electronic equipment, for example bio-resonance and also other aids such as the pendulum and muscle testing. Reaching behind the counter and giving a remedy within two minutes of seeing a patient cannot be described as serious homœopathic treatment. A remedy is then only given according to the name of the disease, and the laws of Classical Homœopathy (individuality, single remedy and dose, etc.) are ignored.

The Complex Remedy

A further attempt to simplify homœopathy is the giving of so-called complex remedies. What does that mean? As the name suggests, it is about mixing different homœopathic substances. Between two and 30(!) remedies in different potencies are mixed. A fever remedy for example is put together from substances that are particularly often used with colds, infections, and fever. The hope is that one of these remedies will be correct.

Complex homœopathy is a thorn in the side to every Classical Homœopath. Hahnemann, Kent, Allen, Hering and whatever the great homœopaths are called, would turn in their graves if they knew what was happening to their bequest. Here again, remedies are given according to the name of the disease, and the laws of Classical Homœopathy are ignored.

Complex remedies are less convincing in the practice. How should the organism know upon what information to react? If one analyzed the mode of action of the individual substances in a complex remedy, one would often see that they cancel each other in their action and act suppressively.

The daily homœopathic practice repeatedly shows us that treatment is more difficult when complex remedies have previously been taken. The body has lost its ability to react after dealing with the flood of information that the complex remedy represents.

A further argument against complex remedies is that in this mixture, there has been no remedy proving on the healthy. So how should one then know how this mixture will act on people? One knows from chemistry that a mixture of two or more substances can have a quite different action than each of the original substances alone.

We do not know the effect of taking several medicines together or the interaction between them. In homœopathy we know the effects of a single remedy, as this has been tested on healthy people.

Only a single appropriate homœopathic remedy will bring into being a lasting cure. Thus the Anthroposophical Medicine according to Rudolf Steiner and the Biochemic System of Medicine according to Schüssler are not Classical Homœopathy, since in both forms of therapy, as a rule, different homœopathic remedies are used simultaneously.

Acute and Chronic Diseases

n homœopathic treatment, one distinguishes between acute and chronic illness. With the acute as with the chronic illness, the Vital Force is disturbed. The power of self-healing seeks relief via the body and the excretory organs.

If these processes of excretion and cleansing such as skin eruptions, diarrhoea, vomiting, sweating, fever, runny nose or eruptions are treated with medicines and are suppressed, acute illness can develop into chronic illness, since the Vital Force is being prevented from bringing the disease to the surface of the body. The organism cannot become healthy in this way. The disease "ulcerates" at a deeper level. If it was an attack of sweating or a cold, the patient will later suffer from, for example, bronchial asthma, joint problems, disturbances of the circulation, vertigo, psychological problems, etc.

Acute diseases

In acute illnesses, the Vital Force of the sick person can, as a rule, conquer the acute situation with its own energy. Health is usually restored of its own accord within a short time.

With the correctly chosen homœopathic remedy, the cure of acute conditions such as anxiety, eye infections, insect bites, diarrhoea, vomiting, coughs, colds, fever, sore throats and ear pain, fear of exams, travel sickness, exhaustion, sunburn, children teething, etc. can be supported.

Similarly, homœopathic remedies are successfully used with injuries such as torn ligaments, bruising, sprains, crushes etc. Not only superficial but also serious injuries that require orthodox medical treatment can be treated with acute remedies, in order to support the healing process.

Chronic diseases

The Vital Force behaves quite differently with chronic conditions. Typically, we find repeated unsuccessful attempts to restore health. On the rarest of occasions do these heal of their own accord. The question here is why is the power of self-healing of the organism too weak to produce a cure? The weakening of the Vital Force through the miasmatic burden (see Chapter: *The Miasmatic Disposition)* as well as through suppression (see Chapter: *Suppression)* creates the most important causes of chronic diseases.

The true strength of Classical Homœopathy is in the treatment of chronic diseases of the psyche and of the body, e.g. fears, nervousness, anxiety, depression, complaints from stress and of being overtaxed, sleeplessness, headaches, vertigo/fainting, muscle and joint pains, allergies, respiratory complaints, infection of the middle ear (otitis media), backache, heart and circulation problems, colds, sinus infections, skin diseases, stomach and intestinal problems, hayfever, kidney-bladder complaints, gynaecological illnesses etc. Also very treatable are developmental, learning and behavioural disturbances in children.

Chronic diseases can only be cured by constitutional therapy that takes account of the whole person (see Chapter: *Constitutional Treatment).*

The Miasmatic Disposition

n connection with the occurrence of chronic diseases or inborn bodily or mental disablement, the miasmatic disposition is of great importance for homœopathic treatment. The subject of miasms is very complex and can only be touched upon in this chapter. You will find a tabular summary at the end of the chapter.

Taking miasms into account permits a much deeper harmonisation of the Vital Force. With this understanding, entirely new perspectives are opened into the treatment of deep-seated illness.

To illustrate:

Every winter your child has weeks of bad coughs. The infections attack not only the bronchi but extend to the ears. The bronchial catarrh or the ear infections are each treated with antibiotics. You do not always want to give these, and therefore you consult a homœopath.

The following autumn, the inevitable recurring cough is treated with the appropriate homœopathic remedy before it ends in bronchitis. Some days later the fuss is over and the child enjoys the best of health. Only, the next cold is already on its way. Again, you go to the homœopath. The cough is, again, successfully treated with a homœopathic remedy.

The young patient is protected from deeper illness. His recurring coughs and ear pains are successfully treated with homœopathic remedies and additional antibiotics can be avoided.

Nevertheless, there remains the question as to why the colds and ear infections occur repeatedly. Clearly the power of self-healing is not sufficient to keep the patient healthy. The actual problem, the weakened immune system, is not being resolved. Even the correctly chosen homœopathic remedy, which was tailored to the acute illness, has not led to a complete cure. The basic weakness, the predisposition to colds, remains.

In all probability, a deeper, inherited disturbance is the cause of this weakness. This disturbance of the Vital Force is known in homœopathy as a "miasm". The miasmatic disposition is often the reason why illness can develop in the organism.

Homœopathic remedies that are not chosen with the miasmatic influence in mind, may defeat the symptoms of disease but not get to the root of the problem, and thus not cure the deeper chronic disease. Treatment with only a view to the current physical symptoms is too superficial. As long as it is only the surface that is being treated one cannot reach the much deeper underlying miasms.

Imagine a fruit tree where one cuts off a withered branch and removes the rotten fruit, and every year one is astonished that the tree provides less fruit and is slowly dying. What causes this tree to be sick? We find rotten roots, changes in the quality of the soil, and that the tree is not getting suitable nourishment. It is sick from the roots up. So it is with humans. The cause of disease lies in the deep, in the roots and not on the periphery.

If the homœopath takes into account the miasmatic viewpoint, he has the possibility of successfully treating even quite deep seated weaknesses.

Thus, taking the patient's medical history and particularly that of the close family and ancestors is of the greatest importance. (See Chapter: Case Taking in the Practice)

All diseases, acute and chronic, our own as well as those of relations, and our character traits, are divided into four miasmatic groups. The basis of all disease is "Psora". Developing from that are the "Sycotic" and "Syphilitic" miasms. Hahnemann had already spoken of these three. Later the "Tubercular" Miasm was added. Through a weakening of the Vital Force the slumbering miasm is awakened. It reveals itself through the symptoms of an illness.

Let us take a closer look at the four miasms.

The Psoric Miasm

Psora is the fundamental miasm. It is the basis for the other miasms. The other miasms can develop from this first weakness. With Psora, functional disturbances occur. They are illnesses without organic changes, in other words, complaints that are a nuisance but not dangerous or life threatening.

Type
External manifestations and characteristics

The typical manifestations of the psoric miasm are skin problems. Since childhood there will have been different forms of skin eruptions, such as eczema, neuro-dermatitis etc. The skin heals poorly and thus gets a dirty appearance.

It causes nervous people that are often troubled by itching. The nervousness is also expressed in a nervous unease, eating hastily, speaking quickly and different tics such as blinking, pulling faces, clearing ones throat etc.

Children are possessive, egotistical; always want to be the centre of attention, cannot share, and always have the feeling of being hard done by. Adults do not show these characteristics quite so obviously.

Triggers
Factors that activate miasms

Skin eruptions and discharges, such as runny nose, sweat, menstruation, diarrhoea etc., are relieving for the psoric miasm. If these are suppressed (see Chapter: *Suppression*) then Psora is activated and new diseases occur at a deeper, psoric level. Illnesses from other miasms may occur, since Psora, of course, prepares the way for new miasmatic illness.

> *A 55 year-old woman came to our practice with head-aches and vertigo. These complaints had troubled her for two years. Since then she had become ever more fearful and nervous. After a thorough discussion it was deter-mined that her headaches, vertigo and the psychological changes had all started since taking hormones for sweats and hot flushes in connection with her meno-pause.*
> *By suppressing the sweating with hormones, psoric relief was made impossible and the psoric miasm spread to a deeper level.*

As previously discussed, the psoric person is very nervous and sensitive. Thus, emotional factors such as annoyance, excitement, fright, worries, jealousy and also stress lead to psoric illnesses.

> *Recently, a young manager came to the practice with skin eruptions on his face. During the consultation it became apparent that his skin is always worse when he feels stressed. Also, for months he has had stomach-aches and disturbed sleep, especially after a hectic day. He then lies in bed and cannot switch off. He often wakes during the night covered in sweat. As he is a type who is very exact and conscientious, he feels under pres-sure when he cannot keep certain promises vis-a-vis his*

co-workers. Since taking on a supervisory role six months before, the complaints have worsened.

When asked about illness in the family, he admitted that for years his mother has suffered from nervous gastro-intestinal problems with diarrhoea, his father has a rather fearful nature and the grandmother on the mother's side had bad eczema.

Here, we clearly see the trigger – stress – which, as a result of inherited family traits, activated an existing psoric miasm.

The Sycotic Miasm

In sycosis we are dealing with illnesses that occur slowly and accompany the patient through the years. The illness expresses itself in the early stages with chronic, sticky secretions, deep-seated catarrh, vaginal infections etc.

In an advanced stage "growths" appear such as warts, cysts, myomas (fatty lumps), knots, also rheumatic and psychological illnesses.

Type

External manifestations and characteristics

The visible signs of sycosis are warts, moles, strawberry marks or port wine stains, oily skin, as well as pronounced hair growth and hair on unwanted places (for example hair growth on women). As a result of chronic sinus infections and regular appearance of polyps the patient speaks nasally. In sycosis, we find acne persisting over many years, leaving deep scarring.

The sycotic person differs from the psoric by appearing rather blocked. He is often stubborn and inflexible. According to the depth of the illness, melancholy, low spirits up to deep depression, can be seen.

Triggers
Factors that activate miasms

Warts, fungal infections as well as the typical yellow green discharges are relieving for the sycotic miasm. Should they be suppressed (see Chapter: *Suppression),* sycosis will be activated and new disease will occur at a deeper, sycotic level.

Because of this disease picture of warts, moles, bony growths, cysts, polyps, crooked nasal passages, myomas, haemorrhoids, hallux etc., these patients are often operated upon. These operations, as with vaccinations, deepen the sycotic miasm, whereby even worse illnesses can develop.

> *A 43 year-old mother of two children sought us out because of rheumatic complaints in the joints of the hand and fingers. These complaints interfered with her work as a nurse and in the home. In order to fulfil her duties she takes anti-inflammatory drugs. From taking a history we find that she had many warts as a child and severe acne during puberty. During her nursing training she suffered from a chronic bladder infection and vaginal fungi (candida). Between her two pregnancies she suffered a miscarriage. As a baby, her daughter had purulent eye infections, and in the son, infections of the sinuses (in the jaw and forehead) have occurred.*
>
> *The patient is concerned about her health, as her mother had polyarthritis with deformed joints. The father recently had to have an operation on his slipped disc. In his youth, he suffered from kidney stones. The grandmother on the father's side had two miscarriages. From this history we see a clear advance in disease with increasing age, as a result of the familial sycotic disposition.*

The Syphilitic Miasm

We find destructive processes in this miasm. Diseases progress very quickly, go deep straight away, and are destructive. To differentiate psora, sycosis and syphilis let us look at the example of skin disease. In psora we have intense itching, possibly with redness, in sycosis continual suppuration and bad scarring, and in syphilis ulcerations leading to "deep craters".

Congenital disturbances, malformations, and birth injuries belong in this group, also addictions such as alcoholism and drug taking. Destructiveness is not only apparent in the body but also in behaviour. Syphilitic people often tend towards violence or mental illness and demonstrate suicidal tendencies. Complaints are worse at night.

Type
External manifestations and characteristics

The syphilitic miasm is easy to recognise. The deformations and malformations such as hair lip, cleft palate, deformation of the jaw, misalignment and deformation of teeth, severe dental caries already in small children etc. point to it.

The syphilitically disposed person often has destructive thoughts, tending towards severe aggression with violence, even to criminal tendencies. This destructiveness is not only directed towards others; it is also aimed at the self in the form of severe addictiveness, extreme mental illnesses, even suicide.

Triggers
Factors that activate miasms

In patients with a strong inherited syphilitic taint, small causes can often result in severe syphilitic disease. A bagatelle is enough to set in motion destructive processes such as, for example, alcohol and drug consumption, deepest depression up to suicide, and severe physical illnesses.

As in no other of the miasms, there is the greatest danger that suppression can significantly compromise the state of health (see Chapter: *Suppression*).

The patient is sitting on a powder keg, so to speak. A "tiny" surgical procedure and the Vital Force is no longer in balance. The illness takes a dramatic turn or a new illness occurs very shortly thereafter.

> *A mother comes with her five-year-old son. She is at her wits end. His extreme temper tantrums are not only directed at his parents but principally against his younger sister and the neighbours' children. Any minor annoyance and he is hitting, biting, and scratching, and whatever he can get his hands on is thrown to the ground and destroyed.*
>
> *In addition, his mother is concerned about his dental caries, severe misalignment of his teeth, a dental enamel defect diagnosed by his dentist, and a mild deformation of the jaw.*
>
> *We learn from the case history that the mother had a heart defect at birth, which was surgically corrected. Some relatives on the father's side had alcohol problems. An uncle had been severely depressed and committed suicide. An aunt has been living for years in a psychiatric clinic and a grandfather had died of Alzheimer's.*
>
> *We can see that this child came into this world with a strong syphilitic taint, which he is already demonstrating at such a young age.*

The Tubercular Miasm

The tubercular miasm is a combination of the psoric and syphilitic miasms. Therefore, we find both psoric and syphilitic traits, i.e. restlessness and nervousness of psora combined with the destructiveness of the syphilitic contribution.

Decades ago, tubercular miasms appeared principally in the form of tuberculosis and rickets. Today, we see the tubercular signs in the form of chronic middle ear infections, angina, and diseases of the airways such as bronchitis, pneumonia and pseudo-croup. Hay fevers and other allergies, on the increase for years, similarly belong to this group.

The energy reserves of the tubercular disposed patient are rapidly exhausted. For days he is full of the need to do things, then suddenly he is overcome by a leaden tiredness that requires a long time to recover from.

Type

External manifestations and characteristics

In the tubercular miasm, there is severe restlessness, hyperactivity, and the need for motion is excessive. This leads to exhaustion, as a result of the constitutional weakness. A tubercular person always wants novelty, is not satisfied with what he has, continually requires stimuli, excitement, thrills, and often seeks danger. He suffers from poor concentration, is easily distracted, is impulsive and tends to have outbursts of temper.

The tubercular disposed person is easy to spot. Typically long and thin, rocketing build, popularly known as a "beanstalk". A narrow chest, or a pigeon chest also points to a tubercular taint. We often see swollen glands in childhood.

Triggers

Factors that activate miasms

As with the sycotically disposed, the tubercular tolerate vaccinations badly. After vaccination latent tubercular miasm breaks out and tubercular complaints develop. With the sycotically disposed, sycotic complaints occur.

As with all miasms, medication and operations have a suppressive effect on the tubercular miasm, leading to the patient becoming ill on a deeper, miasmatic, level. In our practice we often notice that tubercular children are more prone to illness and are regularly prescribed antibiotics. This promotes the tubercular miasm.

> *A 15 year-old girl has suffered for years from a severe allergic asthma, which is badly interfering with her sport. From the age of six months to three years old, she was ill two to three times every winter with middle ear and throat infections. At the age of four, she suffered severe bronchitis. At five, she had to be hospitalised because of pneumonia. These illnesses were treated with antibiotics. In all these years, she was very restless and hyperactive. In primary school she had learning and concentration difficulties. The school psychiatrists diagnosed ADHD. The family history points to a severe tubercular taint. The grandmother and two of her sisters got TB as children, one dying from it. The mother twice had pneumonia and is extremely underweight. The father had been ill with meningitis in his childhood, and his mother and grandmother both had goitre.*
>
> *Already from early childhood the severe tubercular disposition in the relations is demonstrated in this girl in the form of repeated infectious diseases. Through the many medicinal treatments the tubercular miasm settled at a deeper level. Hyperactivity and, later, allergic asthma developed.*

It is often seen in everyday practice that illnesses are markedly multi-miasmatic, i.e. several miasms burden people. For the sake of clarity, we chose particular cases that can be clearly attributed to a single miasm.

For more advanced reading, we include a list of references at the end of the book.

Symptoms

Complaints that appear in the patient or relatives:

Psora	Sycosis	Syphilis	Tubercular
• Fears, e.g. before exams, of the future, of loss	• Mental illnesses such as depression, mania, compulsive neuroses	• Violence, suicidal	• ADHD, hyperactivity, poor concentration, temper tantrums
• Nervousness, great restlessness, stress, nail-biting	• Warts, fatty tumours, moles, polyps	• Addictions: drugs, alcohol, tobacco, narcotics	• Night sweats
• Hot flushes from nerves	• Poorly healing wounds, herpes, fungal infections	• Cerebral disturbances	• Grinding teeth
• Headaches from nerves	• Yellow-green mucous discharges from nose (sinusitis), eye (eye infections in the new-born), ear, lungs, vagina	• Mental handicaps	• Febrile convulsions
• Vertigo from nerves		• Gangrene, ulcers	• Anaemia, tendency to bleeding, nose bleeds
• Burning skin, itching, poor healing, dirty appearance	• Cysts, growths, breast lumps – slow growing	• Deformation of any type: heart, kidneys, ovaries, uterus, face, jaw, teeth, ears, fingernails, toenails, extremities	• Swollen glands (lymph glands, tonsils), glandular fever
		• Stillbirths, sudden infant death (SIDS)	• Chronic otitis media, diminished hearing,

50

• Runny nose, watery, causes sores, irritation of the skin	• Prostate-, vagina-, fallopian tube-inflammations, myomas, miscarriages, growths & deformities	• Osteoporosis, spina bifida (open spine), nightly bone pains (growth pains) and other bone diseases	• Pseudo-croup, bronchitis, pneumonia
• Gastro-intestinal complaints of nervous origins, ravenous, diarrhoea	• Inflammation of bladder and kidney, pelvis	• Multiple sclerosis, muscle-loss, Parkinsonism, epilepsy, Alzheimer's	• Tuberculosis
• Sleep disturbances, difficulty falling asleep from racing thoughts, waking early	• Rheumatism, arthritis, gout, lumbago, chronic back pain	• Down's Syndrome (mongolism), Turner's syndrome	• Rickets
• Hoarseness from nervousness, overstraining the vocal chords	• Hallux, hammer toe, bony growths	• Deafness, deaf & dumb, blindness (congenital)	• Pollen-, animal-, mite-, food-allergies
	• Kidney & bladder stones	• Syphilis, AIDS	• Thyroid disease such as goitre, over-active
	• Varicose veins	• Cancer, rapidly advanced	• Meningitis and its complications
	• Cancers occurring over years		

An incomplete excerpt from specialist scientific literature

Incurable Diseases

No method of healing, not even homœopathy, can perform miracles. Patients who, for years, have suffered severely, have been subjected to many operations and have only managed to live a halfway tolerable life by taking powerful drugs cannot be completely cured – either with homœopathy or any other therapy. The organism is not in a position to regenerate, not even with the assistance of a homœopathic remedy, for example, badly deformed joints, as a result of arthritis and polyarthritis.

There is no homœopathic replacement therapy for a diabetic who has relied on insulin injections for years. An organ that has not been able to function for years can no longer be reactivated. The pancreas is atrophied, and nothing can make it function again. Organ damage, which is also difficult to cure, can occur as a result of years of medication

The therapeutic approach of homœopathy consists in the relief of suffering in the severely ill, and to accompany them in their darkest hour, so that they are calmer, in less pain, and in a better position to accept their situation. By strengthening the will to live and the Vital Force, drugs can often be reduced and side effects made to disappear.

An example:

Mrs H., 50 years old, has suffered from severe polyarthritis with deformed joints for years. She depends on the daily consumption of cortisone. Some months earlier she had a severe rheumatic attack. The dose of cortisone had to be increased. Her blood sugar levels increased shortly thereafter. Diabetes was diagnosed and the lady had to take additional medication for that.

This lady could be helped with homœopathy and a change in her diet to such an extent that her consultant was able to establish during her next follow-up that her sugar levels were normal again. The additional medication was withdrawn and the cortisone greatly reduced.

Further factors that can hinder a cure, or make it more difficult, are very demanding family situations that one cannot escape from. Poor life-style choices, which the patient cannot or will not give up, can hinder a cure, such as a gross faulty diet, alcohol-, cigarette- or drug-consumption, extreme lack of sleep etc.

Mind you, very often, it can be seen that constitutional treatment gives the patient, over time, much more willpower. He recovers his equilibrium and the power to work on improving those lifestyle choices that are detrimental to his health.

The Homœopathic Aggravation

A Healing Response

During homœopathic treatment and especially in chronic cases, it is not uncommon that the complaints are temporarily intensified. Old symptoms that one has not experienced for years can, for a short while, re-surface. This means that the symptoms were not cured. Sometimes, these reactions run their course unnoticed, i. e. the patient notices no aggravation, but that doesn't mean that the homœopathic remedy is not working.

These curative reactions are to be viewed positively and demonstrate that the Vital Force has reacted well, the weak points in the body have been located, and the healing process is in motion. Upon taking a remedy, a reaction can occur within two minutes or after some weeks; sometimes after months. The course of events is different for each patient, depending on the remedy given, potency, and the constitution of the patient.

The nature of the curative reaction is unique. If several individuals are given the same remedy in the same potency, they can all react differently, each according to their suscepti-bility and constitution. Often the body reacts by an increase in secretions such as mucous, diarrhoea, nosebleeds, sweats, vaginal discharges etc. Every reaction acts like a pressure valve and represents a sort of self-purification. The organism can find relief and the patient subsequently feels better.

An aggravation is never as bad as the original illness. When, for example, otitis media occurs because of a homœo-pathic remedy, the organism is already strengthened by the remedy. Therefore the course of the illness is less intense and heals quicker.

Reactions are also to be expected on the mental plane. Introverted and blocked people can become temporarily more emotional. If they were previously diplomatic and outwardly stable, they possibly lose patience more quickly, are more irritable, and sometimes explosive. Suppressed experiences surface, are relived, worked upon and dealt with.

The patient begins to get hold of himself. He is better able to deal with expectations placed on him and is less stressed. If before he always wanted to please everyone and couldn't say no, he now guards against this tendency. The patient is also better able to deal with his emotions, feels more at ease, more stable and free.

Sometimes, the patient finds it difficult to understand certain changes. He requires patience to see these reactions through, but will feel more at ease and strengthened afterwards. Once the healing process is in motion, it must not be interrupted. It is important not to suppress these miscellaneous reactions with medication.

Furthermore, additional homœopathic remedies can disturb this process. Many homœopathic remedies are not compatible with each other and one could cancel the action of the other. As a general rule, one should not take other homœopathic remedies during treatment without the knowledge of the treating homœopath.

Patients with severe organic diseases (asthma, heart disease, diabetes etc.), who have had to take medication over a longer period, naturally continue to take their usual medication. Abrupt cessation would be dangerous. If you have any questions, please consult your homœopath.

To finish, a few examples of possible aggravations:

- angry, irritated, tearful
- intensive dreams
- sweating
- tiredness
- increased menstruation, changes in cycle
- diarrhoea and vomiting
- increased skin eruptions, itching
- head, back, and joint pain
- return of old symptoms

The Healing Process

Hering's law of cure

The question is often put to us: "how long will this course of healing take?" The time taken to achieve a cure is dependent on many factors. Each case of illness is individual, and everyone reacts uniquely.

A general rule on treatment duration, therefore, does not exist. Cure can occur immediately or require quite some time. An illness that occurs suddenly and developed quickly is fundamentally cured quicker than one that slowly creeps up on us.

One must also be mindful of how deep the particular disturbance lies, and how far it has spread throughout the organism. Should serious changes have occurred in the organs or tissues, it takes longer for the Vital Force to complete its "clean-up" work.

Young people and children react, as a rule, faster than older people. Patients who have taken a lot of medication or experienced a multitude of different therapies are often not capable of reacting adequately to homœopathic remedies.

The duration of the illness, as well as inherited suscep-tibility (miasmatic disposition), also plays an important part.

The dialogue with the patient is also of importance. It is not enough, after taking a thorough case history, to simply give the patient a couple of globules and say "see you again in one month". It is important that the homœopath understands the patient and can demonstrate and explain the context and origins of the history of his illness. As soon as the patient bet-ter understands his symptoms he will also be more receptive to the various reactions caused by the homœopathic remedy.

One is continually confronted with patients who, after years of unsuccessful treatment with various therapies, expect a cure within weeks from homœopathy. Should this not happen, they turn, disappointed, to a new therapeutic modality.

Remember, chronic disease develops over years and is deep in the organism. The Vital Force must be addressed and brought on the correct course. That often requires patience. Give your organism the time it requires to become truly healthy.

A cure can be made difficult or impossible by the lifestyle of the patient, such as an over-generous consumption of alcohol, smoking, excessive stress, lack of exercise and other health threatening habits, such as drugs, lack of sleep, and poor diet. Also an intolerable family situation can impede or even make a cure impossible.

> *Recently, a businessman came to the practice, who wanted to be relieved of his symptoms of stress using homœopathy. During the consultation he mentioned that his life consisted solely of work. He now expects from homœopathy, thanks to which he is now free of complaints, that he can continue his life with little exercise and sleep, an unhealthy diet and a generous consumption of alcohol.*
>
> *Homœopathic treatment can indeed temporarily cure stress induced complaints. But if the person does not change their unhealthy lifestyle, their complaints will return sooner or later.*

As previously mentioned, there are no general rules for the time required to achieve a cure. The nature of the curative process is subject to laws named after their discoverer Constantine Hering (1802–1880).

He postulated the following three laws of cure:
"The direction of cure occurs
1. From above to below,
2. from within to the outside, and
3. in reverse order to their appearance."

Exactly what is to be understood by this, we will clarify in the following examples:

Hering's 1st law:
From above to below

A patient presents for treatment with a shoulder pain that he has had four months. At the next consultation he is struck by low back pain. "How is your shoulder?" "I no longer feel any pain there". The disease process has moved lower, from the shoulder to the small of the back. Three weeks later, he complains of knee pain. The back, in the meantime, is pain-free. Later he requests a remedy for ankle pain.
We clearly see a transfer of the complaint from above to below.

If one were to give, in ignorance of the law of cure and its healing process, a remedy for the ankle pain, then the patient is freed of his complaint for a short while. But the course of the cure would be suppressed and the old shoulder pains would reoccur.

One must always follow the holistic option of constitutional treatment. The complaints have changed location according to Hering's law. They have transferred from above to below.

As with the back and knee pain, the patient gets no remedy for the new acute condition. After some time he is also free of his ankle pain.

Hering's 2nd law:
From within to the outside

The cure proceeds from the centre to the periphery, i. e. from the important organs to the less important. The mood, the psyche as the "innermost" layer of a person improves first. Afterwards, the vital organs such as heart, liver, kidneys, lungs, and then the locomotor apparatus are healed.

The skin, as the outermost organism, is last to be cured. As the outermost "layer" it performs a cleansing function and as such acts as a valve. Therefore, skin complaints can be very stubborn.

> *A 14 year-old girl regularly suffers from a violent migraine. Often, she must skip school and leave classes prematurely. She takes teasing and conflict with her peers very personally. She often feels that she is not accepted. After a thorough case history she receives her constitutional remedy. At the follow-up consultation one month later, she reported that her migraines occur much more seldom and are less intense. Additionally, she had found a circle of friends. She was very concerned with the warts on her hands, which had greatly increased in the last few months. This case clearly demonstrates the progression of cure from inside to surface. The strengthened organism brings the disease process to the surface via the warts. The psyche is stronger, the headaches better. No remedy was dispensed as the curative process was already underway. After two months the migraines and the warts had completely disappeared.*

Hering's 3rd Law:
In reverse order to their appearance

Illnesses that have recently occurred are healed first. The history of illness will often be rolled back chronologically. Finally, the illnesses one has had the longest disappear.

> *A patient has had sinusitis since childhood, vaginal fungal infection for the last five years, and a severe menstrual complaint for the last year. Thus, the menstrual complaint is the first to be cured, then the vaginal infection, and finally the sinusitis.*

With regard to Hering's law, it is sufficient for only one law to apply in order to speak of a positive healing process.

60

Suppression

Making matters worse

True cure does not just mean the disappearance of symptoms of disease (see Chapter: *Disease and Cure*). As a result of treatment, complaints will often disappear, only to reoccur after a brief while. Here we are thinking of, for example, recurrent cystitis, colds, candida, eczema etc.

Admittedly, medication has made the symptoms disappear. The disease is, however, not cured, since it always returns. The susceptibility is not yet removed. Should the body continually have the energy, despite suppressive treatment, to bring to the fore the same symptoms, this points to a relatively strong Vital Force. With great certainty it repeatedly chooses to produce those symptoms which help it to restore balance.

It is more problematic when, instead of the old complaints, a "new" illness occurs. This illness is often seen as quite independent and not seen in connection with the first. In fact, the basic illness is the same. It has only changed its appearance, i. e. other complaints are making themselves felt.

There is the tendency for the illness to move from the outside surface of the body inwards, and in doing so it becomes more dangerous. This process is called "suppression". It occurs when an illness is treated purely on a symptomatic level, without taking into account the cause – the weakened Vital Force. This suppressive and symptomatic treatment is especially ingrained in orthodox medical thought.

There are different types of suppression:

1. Suppression by Orthodox Medication

The patient has been suffering for a long time with a skin eruption on the hands. He gets a "mild" cortisone-containing ointment from the dermatologist. After a week the skin is healed and the patient is pleased that he is free of this problem so quickly. After three weeks, he gets a severe eruption on his face, hands and back of the knees. He gets a stronger ointment. After six months treatment the skin eruption is finally conquered. The patient forgets the whole affair. Three months later his GP diagnoses elevated blood pressure.

This high blood pressure is a result of the suppression of the skin eruption. It was simply dealt with "cosmetically" i.e. treated superficially, but the root of the illness was not treated. Thus, the disease process moved inwards. During correct homœopathic treatment the skin eruption would first reappear and then the high blood pressure would disappear.

Let us take the example of common influenza. During a viral infection the body temperature, as a rule, rises a few degrees. The immune defences are in full swing. Should the fever be lowered by medication, the patient can go about his daily duties. From a medical viewpoint, the patient is healthy. Only, a few days later the patient feels lethargic, complains of head-, stomach-, and joint-pains. Haven't we all known the following "I have not been well since having the flu"?

Should the patient now come to the practice and be treated with a homœopathic remedy that is selected according to his individual symptoms, in all likelihood the fever will return and sweats will break out.

What has happened? The homœopathic remedy has stimulated the Vital Force, which now seeks the appropriate means to cure the organism. After this healing reaction the patient rapidly feels healthy and ready to take on any new challenges.

2. Suppression by Homœopathic Remedies

One can also suppress with homœopathy and other modes of treatment if a person is not seen in his entirety. The danger of suppression is very great, particularly with homœopathic complex remedies, in which single components are chosen according to the disease symptoms. Matters are also made worse when the patient's individual symptomatology is not taken into account.

The same problem occurs when one uses homœopathic single remedies according to the name of the disease. Especially colds and allergic diseases such as hayfever are then homœopathically suppressed.

Recently, a mother and her six-year-old son came as an emergency to the practice. For days he had had a severe cough, with night-time worsening to the point of vomiting. What had happened?

Three weeks ago, the little boy came home from a school trip with burning eyes and a heavy nasal discharge. The mother went to the nearest chemist and got the homœopathic remedy Allium cepa for the hayfever symptoms, which she gave to him three times a day. The symptoms worsened and a hayfever complex remedy was given.

One week later, the little boy was additionally given the homœopathic remedy Bryonia for his cough, which he took for several days.

The disease process had moved into bronchitis, as a result of the organ orientated approach and remedy prescriptions for the hayfever symptoms.

Every homœopath must observe during the treatmen whether the complaint that the patient came with is truly cured or just suppressed. Often, it is believed that one canno suppress using homœopathic remedies. However, this is false Even in acute cases, the observation of the totality of the patient is vitally important.

3. Suppression of the Course of the Cure

Patients are continually mentioning during case taking that they are currently receiving other therapies such as Bach Flower Remedies, Schüssler biochemical salts, bio resonance, acupuncture, reflexology, etc.

An example:

> Based on the totality of his symptoms, a patient with nervous digestive disturbances and problems sleeping gets the homœopathic remedy Lycopodium in the 1M potency. After a few weeks, he notices an improvement in the digestive tract. Also his sleep is better again. However, back pains that he had had earlier, and that represent a reaction to the homœopathic remedy, now trouble him. The patient feels that this complaint is irksome and sees an acupuncturist, who treats his back and removes the pains in a short period of time. Short-ly thereafter, the stomach complaints reoccur. He is nervous again and has renewed sleep disturbances.
> Here the harmonious curative process was disturbed. The disease moved from the superficial (back) inwards (nerves, stomach). It will now take longer for the or ganism and the healing process to be brought back on track again.

It is well known that "too many cooks spoil the broth" and differing therapies disturb the harmonious healing pro cess. The organism is overburdened by different influences an information and no longer knows which stimulus to react to. Various reactions may occur during the homœopathic healing process. Should these then be treated by other therapies, which may act suppressively, the healing process will be disturbed. After an explanatory chat, the patient must choose a particular therapy which he should then stick to. Only then has the body the chance to react optimally.

> *A six-year-old boy came to the practice because of bedwetting. He also has suffered from a purulent severe sore throat with high temperature two to three times a year. This is treated by his paediatrician. After a thorough study of the case history we prescribed a constitutional remedy, whereupon his bedwetting ceased. Later, he complained of a severe sore throat and the mother gave him a remedy from the home medicine cupboard, and his sore throat improved. At the follow-up weeks later, the mother complained that her son had been wetting the bed again. This started two days after the sore throat and was a regular occurrence again.*
>
> *Using the homœopathic remedy from the medicine cupboard, the sore throat was treated and consequently suppressed. The healing process was thus disturbed and the chronic complaint, the bedwetting, reoccurred.*

This case clearly shows the suppressive effect of the acute homœopathic remedy on the deeper acting constitutional remedy.

During homœopathic constitutional treatment no other homœopathic remedy should be taken without consulting the treating homœopath. Only he or she knows the context of the entire case and can appropriately judge the course of the cure.

Orthodox medicine that is taken for complaints which appear during constitutional treatment can also suppress the healing process. For this reason, the taking of such medication should be agreed with the homœopath.

Case-taking in the Practice

Getting all the facts

I n the previous chapters, we have discussed the theoretical basis of Classical Homœopathy. We now want to show how this is used in the practice.

Investigations

Before the first consultation, a patient should find out about the nature of any illnesses existing within the family (see Chapter: *The Miasmatic Disposition*). This is not always easy and requires much goodwill and persistence in order to get relatives to reveal their history of illnesses. Parents often haven't taken much notice of illnesses, are no longer aware of them, or do not wish to talk about the past.

The more detailed a patient's knowledge of the family history, the simpler the consultation. The homœopath gets important information on the miasmatic influences of the case and the homœopathic remedies to be considered.

It is important to know which illnesses parents, grandparents, great-grandparents, uncles, aunts, siblings and children have suffered from. Operations and the cause of death of relatives are also of importance.

- Cancer
- Tuberculosis
- Diabetes type 1 and type 2
- Rheumatism
- Polyarthritis
- Alcoholism
- Depression
- Suicide
- Arthritis

- Gout
- Varicose veins
- Ulcers
- Strokes
- Paralysis
- Heart disease
- Growths
- Premature births, miscarriages

- Stillbirths
- Skin diseases
- Deformities
- Blood diseases
- Lung diseases

- Sexual diseases
- Infectious diseases
- Vaccination damage
- Allergies
- etc.

Furthermore, the patient needs to list his own illnesses, significant operations and life events in chronological order. The homœopath also needs to know about medication that was taken in the past or is being taken now.

Additionally for children, the following information is important.

- Course of the pregnancy
- Any medication taken by the mother during pregnancy
- The course of delivery
- Size and weight of the newborn
- Appearance
- Defects
- Birth damage
- Breast-fed, how long?
- Feeding behaviour
- Development, teething, walking, speech
- Vaccinations, dates and possible reactions
- Any other information the mother can give.

Case history

Taking a patient's case begins with the first contact in the waiting room. That first impression often speaks volumes. How is his manner, his handshake, is he nervous, tense, or is he at ease?

There then follows a long discussion about his actual complaints such as:

- Location
- Where it began
- Cause
- Times when free of the complaint
- Characteristics of the pain
- Factors that worsen,
- Factors that make better
- Accompanying symptoms of the main complaint
- Changes in mood during the complaint
- etc.

For a complete case history, all aspects of the patient must be noted. Therefore, other details about body and mind are extremely important. For example:

- Other complaints
- Sleep/dreams
- Gastro-intestinal symptoms
- Menstruation
- Temperature regulation
- Sweating
- Fears, worries, sadness
- Self-confidence
- Insults, injured feelings
- Temperament
- Family situation
- etc.

Not only are the current mental and physical state of importance but also the complete biography of the patient from childhood to the present day. The homœopath attempts to record and understand the person in his entirety. While taking the case, it is important to search for the cause of an illness, whether physical or mental in nature, no matter how long ago it occurred. The cause could have taken its hold already in childhood.

This chapter attempts to be a brief insight into case taking. It is not a conclusive listing of all the useful information that is gathered. In the homœopathic practice, case taking is more comprehensive. All this collected information gives the most complete picture possible of the patient. It is akin to putting single mosaic tiles together to form a picture. The more tiles available, the clearer the picture. Only then can the homœopath decide with which remedy the patient should be treated.

Constitutional Treatment

Treating the whole you

n the previous chapters, we have illuminated various aspects of homœopathy. All of these are taken into account and utilised in homœopathic constitutional treatment. You will see from the following case history the complexity of homœopathy and the procedures for treating a chronic illness.

> *Mrs H., 52 years, came for a variety of complaints. Firstly, she reported rheumatic pains in both shoulders with circulation and sensory disturbances down both arms, especially in the hands. She wakes in the night because of it. For years she has suffered from a recurrent lower back and hip pain, which is disabling. The shoulder pain from which she has suffered since the age of 37, has worsened to such an extent in the last five months that her rheumatologist prescribed some cortisone injections and strong anti-rheumatics.*

So much for the first spontaneous report from the patient. The mere description of these symptoms however, is not sufficient for a homœopathic prescription. The patient must be understood in her totality in order to arrive at the correct remedy.

> *From the question of whether she has any other complaints, she tells that since the age of 20 she has always had recurring severe cystitis and for years has had to be treated for sinusitis every winter. In the last few years, she has greatly increased in weight and suffers terribly because of it.*

So much for the patient's current bodily problems.

Homœopathy views people as a unity of body, mind and soul. Separation of this whole is impossible. The character and mood of the patient plays a vital role in ascertaining the correct homœopathic remedy.

> *She describes herself as a woman with a great sense of duty. She has always looked after others, been there only for her two, now grown-up, children and her husband, often felt guilty and couldn't say no. She cannot forgive herself for an abortion she had at the age of 36.*
>
> *Now she is under pressure from her mother, who is in need of care. Indeed, she speaks of psychological terror, against which she cannot defend herself. On speaking of her childhood, she begins to cry and explains that she was an unwanted child and had done all she could to not be a burden to her parents, and to be loved.*

Further, the following history is taken from the questionnaire filled out by the patient:

Age	illness/operation
7	various warts removed
8	measles, pneumonia
9–18	severe sore throats 1–2 times per year
19	appendectomy
20–today	cystitis
23	miscarriage in the third month
26	salpingitis (inflammation of fallopian tubes)
28	Caesarean section
28–today	depression
31	growths operated
35	nervous breakdown
36	abortion
37	colon polyps operated
37	myoma, cysts operated
37–today	shoulder, back pain
38–today	chronic sinusitis

50	warts, fatty tumours operated
3 months later	6 weeks severe bleeding, followed by the menopause
50 – today	severe rheumatic phases

Each illness was treated with the corresponding orthodox medication.

The key question is – what was the reason for the rheumatic shoulder complaints appearing at the age of 37? The abortion at 36 had weakened the Vital Force as a result of the great mental and physical stress. Following that, the lady had severe colic and the colon polyps were operated on. Subsequently, heavy bleeding started, whereby the myoma and various cysts were operated on. As a result of all this suppression, the illness now manifests itself in a rheumatic form.

The operation on the warts and fatty tumours at 50 years of age and the subsequent, hormonally treated, severe bleeding acted further suppressively. After that, the menopause occurred, for which she received another hormonal preparation, which she continues to take. Subsequently, the rheumatic complaints dramatically worsened.

Here one can clearly see that, after the removal of the warts and tumours, the organism sought a new outlet for its disturbance in the form of heavy bleeding. The hormonal treatment stopped the bleeding and the disease process moved to a deeper level (see Chapter: *Suppression*).

From the questionnaire we get the following family history:

Mother's side:

Mother	two miscarriages, varicose veins operated several times
Uncle	kidney stones
Aunt	cysts operated on, depression
Grandmother	gout, miscarriage
Grandfather	cancer

Father's side:

Father	Operations on prostate
Uncle	gall-stones, hernia (hiatus)
Grandmother	operations on intestines
Grandfather	rheumatism

Son	hernia/rupture
Daughter	chronic colds

We see a clear sycotic influence from the family history. The illnesses of the patient also belong to the sycotic miasm. For more details, please see Chapter: *The Miasmatic Disposition*.

After a thorough study and evaluation of all these facts, the homœopath prescribes a constitutional remedy. Reactions and the healing process must now be carefully observed.

> *At the subsequent follow-ups, the patient tells us that her menstruation, which had ceased two years ago, has returned and is very heavy. The shoulder pains have disappeared, but her hip and back pains are worse. This disturbs her much less than the previous shoulder pain with the associated lack of sensation and sleep disturbances.*
>
> *She further reports that she had cried at the beginning, and old issues had resurfaced. This had unburdened her. Additionally, her husband and children noticed that she is not such a pushover any more. She also has more contact with other women, which is very rewarding. As an aside, she remarks on how she has lost some weight. For almost two years, she had irregular periods. The hip pains are much better. Sometimes she still notices the joint. The complaints are tolerable, and psychologically she is much more balanced and full of a positive outlook on life.*

This case clearly shows the reaction of the Vital Force to the homœopathic remedy. The organism finds relief in the heavy bleeding and the shoulder pain disappears. As soon as the body no longer requires this pressure valve, the bleeding stops of its own accord, which is normal at the age of 52.

In accordance with Hering's law (see Chapter: *Direction of Cure*) the complaints go from above to below, in this case from shoulder to the hips.

Also of importance is that this woman has become mentally much stronger, can resolve her worries, is more open and independent, and was able to build a new circle of friends. In the course of the two years treatment, the condition of the patient had improved to such an extent that she was able to lead an almost complaint-free life.

It should be mentioned that the patient must, in future, take heed of the signs from her body. The organism had shown that it reacted very sensitively to obvious suppressions. As soon as any problems reoccur, these should be viewed afresh in their totality and treated with the appropriate homœopathic remedy.

In this example, the patient received the same homœopathic remedy at infrequent internals. It is often seen in practice, though, that several homœopathic remedies are required over longer periods of time when treating chronic disease. In this chapter, we have given you a little insight into the work and thought processes of the homœopath.

Homœopathy during Pregnancy

Pregnancy is a special stage in the life of a woman. It also represents a stress on the female organism. If the pregnant woman disposes of a strong Vital Force she will blossom during this time. If the Vital Force is not so strong then the slumbering chronic miasmatic tendencies surface. Earlier health problems worsen or new symptoms appear.

> Severe "morning" sickness, bloating,
> bleeding, constipation, haemorrhoids, eczema,
> cardiovascular disturbances, nervousness,
> herpes, anaemia, back and joint pains,
> sleep disturbances, vaginal infections etc.,
> are complaints that can often occur.

As many pharmacological substances pass through the placenta, medication often poses a threat to the unborn.

From this point of view, Classical Homœopathy is an invaluable help during pregnancy, birth, and the time thereafter. Correct and appropriate use presents no danger of side effects to mother or child.

The health of the mother is decisive for the development of the foetus. Often one can see in practice, how women who have constitutional treatment before and during the pregnancy encounter their "motherly joy" much easier than in previous pregnancies. There are fewer complications during the birth and they produce healthier children. Various homœopathic remedies are available for the birth preparations. As with all patients, the appropriate remedy is prescribed according to individual symptoms. In this connection it should be mentioned that, increasingly, midwives have some homœopathic knowledge and employ the remedies with great success.

Not only can homœopathic remedies be of assistance during pregnancy and birth, but also mother and child can be helped in the time afterwards. Mastitis is one of the most common problems during breast-feeding. Using appropriate homœopathic treatment, other medication can be avoided. A cure is rapidly achieved and the mother can breast-feed again.

Problems of the involution of the uterus and postnatal depression are also treatable homœopathically.

Homœopathy
for Children

Homœopathic treatment is not only capable of improving the health of babies and young children, but also plays a significant part in our children developing into healthy adults.

It never ceases to astonish how, without a care, our young children are stuffed full with medication. Many mothers seek to avoid medicines during pregnancy. No sooner is the child born and these good resolutions are forgotten. A persistent cough is treated with syrup, skin eruptions suppressed with ointments, fevers controlled with suppositories, and ear pain treated with antibiotics.

As a result of these suppressive actions, the youthful organism cannot build its immune defences sufficiently. It is extraordinarily important that the defensive force is always exercised. Only in this way does the body learn to defend itself and is not helpless and unprotected when exposed to external influences (see Chapter: *Suppression*).

Homœopathic remedies strengthen the immune system and the organism can deal with the illness itself.

Sometimes it happens that, already in their first days and weeks, the newborn have health problems such as conjunctivitis, eczema, nappy rash, digestive problems, vomiting, breathing problems, etc. These early occurring complaints are often a case of miasmatic taint (see Chapter *The Miasmatic Disposition*). Homœopathic treatment protects the child from later, deeper disturbances.

Children often suffer from skin eruptions. These eruptions are to be understood as a defensive response of the Vital Force. It is the result of an inner disturbance of health, manifesting itself on the surface. The body attempts to eliminate the stressful substance via the eliminative organ, the skin. If this process is not recognised and allowed to proceed and the symptoms are treated with medication, then the organism moves the disease process inwards (see Chapter *Suppression*).

When skin eruptions are suppressed, problems with the airways are frequently observed. If an asthmatic child is treated homœopathically, the skin eruptions will occur again for some time. In this way, the lungs are immediately relieved. The illness is being treated at its roots and, after a while, the child returns to complete health.

Homœopathy is capable of treating a broad spectrum of diseases such as:

> three-month cramps, teething problems,
> developmental problems, learning difficulties,
> shyness, fears, stammers, home sickness,
> bedwetting, difficulties with relationships,
> aggression, restlessness, hyperactivity,
> ear infections, sore throats, otitis media,
> mumps, measles, German measles, scarlet fever,
> coughs, hayfever, skin eruptions, etc.

We should not forget that in the initial months, the mother's milk is invaluable. It contains all the vital nourishment and also antibodies, which build the immune system and immune defences of the child, protecting from illness. Breastfed children are in better general health and less prone to disease.

Relaxed surroundings are very important for a sick child. Overanxious parents can hardly radiate the calm that is required for a child's rapid recovery. It is, therefore, very important for the parents to have faith in the self-healing powers of the child and not to panic at every sign of a temperature or cough. Often parents also have to be treated themselves so that their children can recover.

Homœopathy and Sport

Sport is enjoying ever-greater popularity and contributes, when carried out within sensible limits, to a healthy sense of well-being, both at competitive as well as amateur levels. Conditions occurring in connection with sporting activities are eminently treatable with homœopathic remedies.

Sport injuries such as:

sprains, strains, bruising,
inflammation of the joints, complaints
from overuse, also heat stroke,
sunstroke, headaches, cramps, stage fright,
gastro-intestinal problems, colds etc.

are some examples of the therapeutic possibilities. However, homœopathy is not only useful in external injuries. It can also help when orthodox medicine has no answer, for example when a sportsman cannot translate his talent into competitiveness, i.e. is a world champion in training but fails in the competition. Many athletes can perform at their best, but are then suddenly blocked. They are medically examined and are organically found completely healthy. In such instances, the correctly chosen homœopathic remedy helps.

Sports people may be athletically in top condition, but often lack the necessary powers of concentration. This not only hinders their performance, but also increases the risk of injury, since coordination and reactions are no longer optimal. Internal tensions develop, and not infrequently muscle cramps. Homœopathy can help in such cases. For competitive and amateur sports people alike, the more relaxed they are, the better their performance.

In cases where orthodox medical assistance is unavoidable, for example broken bones, Classical Homœopathy can support optimal healing. Healing occurs faster with fewer complications and less pain. The mental state of the patient improves. All these benefits mean that the athlete can begin training again as early as possible.

With correct usage, homœopathic remedies, in contrast to many chemical "wonder drugs", cause no undesired side-effects. This is a great advantage with a view to future health.

Homœopathic
Self-treatment

Ever more people are becoming interested in homœopathy and want to heal minor complaints with homœopathic remedies. Self-medication of simple everyday problems can certainly be useful, but not all complaints are suited to self-treatment.

As you will have noticed while reading the previous chapters, homœopathy is a comprehensive and difficult science that can only be practised after a long and intensive course of studies. The homœopathic first-aid kit cannot under any circumstances replace the visit to the homœopath or doctor. It can, however, perform a valuable service in the treatment of non-dangerous and acute complaints such as:

> colds, fever, influenza,
> gastro-intestinal complaints, insect bites,
> inflammation of the eye, sore throats,
> acute injuries, earache, sunburn, cystitis,
> toothaches, etc.

Chronic or recurrent complaints are not suited to self-treatment. These must be treated by a homœopath using deep acting remedies. With self-medication, one should bear in mind that the organism, as a rule, has enough power to heal itself of minor indispositions. It is important not to turn to the homœopathic first-aid kit for every minor incident. Simpler household remedies such as compresses, baths, herbal teas etc. are often enough to support the Vital Force.

During the course of ongoing homœopathic treatment, the homœopathic first-aid kit should not be used without consulting the homœopath. Otherwise, the curative action of a constitutional remedy could be disturbed and suppressed (see Chapter: *Suppression)*. Furthermore, not all homœopathic remedies are compatible. For emergencies it is useful to have a selection of homœopathic remedies at home, and, after consulting your homœopath, have the appropriate remedy immediately to hand.

A thorough case-taking is very important in finding the homœopathic acute remedy. It consists of a comprehensive observation of the case, as the following example illustrates:

- **Nature of the illness:** diarrhoea, vomiting, fever, insect bites ...
- **Appearance:** pale, red, swollen ...
- **Cause:** injury, food, overheating, cold, stress ...
- **Behaviour of the patient:** apathetic, fearful, excited ...
- **Sensations of the patient:** nature of the pain (throbbing, sticking, etc.) cold and shivering, itching ...
- **Modalities** (factors that makes the complaint better or worse): heat, cold, resting, movement time of day ...

In order to acquire some confidence in the choice of the most suitable acute remedy, it is a good idea to attend a homœopathic first-aid course (information available from the translator).

Homœopathic first-aid kits are manufactured by Helios Homœopathic Pharmacy and are available directly from Helios (see the Bibliography Section for the address), other homœopathic pharmacies, or from the translator.

Taking your Medicine

There are several points to observe when taking the remedy that will contribute to the success of the treatment:

- Do not to touch the homœopathic remedies with your hands.
- Store them well away from strong-smelling substances.
- Do not expose the remedy to extreme heat or sunlight.
- Do not smoke, eat or drink for 30 minutes before and after taking the remedy.
- Let the remedy slowly dissolve in the mouth and only take it with a completely clean mouth; never directly after brushing your teeth.
- Completely avoid the use of camphor and substances containing camphor, for example Vick VapoRub, and other strong smelling oils. Also do not rub others with them. Otherwise, the action of homœopathic remedies can be cancelled or considerably weakened.
- During the course of constitutional treatment, no other homœopathic remedy should be taken without consulting your homœopath.
- Regular consumption of black tea, coffee, Cola, peppermints, and Camilla tea is to be avoided. Cereal coffee has proven to be a good substitute for coffee. For example, Bambu Coffee Substitute from Bioforce, or Caro from Nestlé.

Questions
and Answers (FAQ)

Q: *I am always getting cystitis and my doctor continually finds bacteria in my urine. I have had enough of the antibiotics taken over the years. Is there a homœopathic remedy for these bacteria?*

A: No, homœopathy has no remedy against these bacteria. Nevertheless, chronic or recurrent cystitis can be treated very well constitutionally, since foreign germs only nest and cause damage in a weak organism. Your body's defensive powers must be strengthened and then you will be free from illnesses for the most part.

Q: *We have adopted a child and want it to receive constitutional treatment. Unfortunately we do not know of her miasmatic background. Despite this, is it possible to treat our child homœopathically?*

A: Yes, your child can be treated. It would be better to know the family miasmatic background, but the predispositions will be apparent in the child. A particularly thorough case history will be important here.

Q: *My two-year-old child found the homœopathic first-aid kit, some of the tubes have been opened and all the globules swallowed. Must I reckon with signs of poisoning and other reactions?*

A: No, you don't need to worry. There won't be a reaction whether your child has taken only two globules or the whole bottle. You would only expect to see a reaction if your child were to take a couple of globules at regular internals.

Q: *My homœopath is rather critical towards vaccinations. My paediatrician has another opinion and approves of all vaccinations. Where can I find a critical discussion of the pros and cons of vaccinations?*

A: You can find comprehensive information on this subject by sending a SAE to: The Informed Parent, PO Box 870, Harrow, Middlesex HA3 7UW, Tel. 020-8861-1022, www.informedparent.co.uk. See also the book by Trevor Gunn: Mass Immunisation. A point in question, or Susan Curtis's book: A Handbook of Homœopathic Alternatives to immunisation.

Q: *I have heart disease and have been dependent on medication for many years. I would like to have my chronic back pain and headaches treated homœopathically. But a colleague at work has said that this is not possible as long as I am taking my medication. Homœopathy only works when no orthodox medication is being taken.*

A: This is not the case. Unfortunately, this misconception is still doing the rounds. Homœopathic treatment can definitely help you. A sudden cessation of medication would be absolutely irresponsible and dangerous. Homœopathic remedies work on a different level and can still work even when taking orthodox medical drugs.

Q: *I have to have an operation in the near future. Is there any point in starting homœopathic treatment now?*

A: The question is, when is the operation? If there is sufficient time before the operation, it would be best to have constitutional treatment. Someone who has had constitutional strengthening before an operation will tolerate it better.

The powers of self-healing are increased and convalescence proceeds faster. Should the date be imminent, the homœopath treats the respective symptoms before and after the operation. Problems such as a fear of the operation, nausea after the anaesthetic, pain, poor healing of the wounds, etc. respond well to the appropriate homœopathic remedies.

Q: *My homœopath has given me Sepia for violent period pains. It has helped a lot. Now I have passed this tip on to my friend, but her period pains are no better.*

A: Sepia is a deep acting constitutional remedy that was prescribed by your homœopath on the basis of the totality of your symptoms and not just for the period pains.

Viewing each patient as a unique individual is an important fundamental law in homœopathy. Each person becomes sick in their own specific way and produces their own disease symptoms and the most suitable remedy for them, and them alone, must be found. The remedy that helped you need not also be the specific remedy for your friend.

Q: *I was prescribed Arsenicum album 200C by my homœopath. This troubled me since arsenic is known to be very poisonous.*

A: You can rest assured. From the 12c potency onwards, there are no longer any molecules of the original drugs. This means the substance is no longer poisonous.

Q: *Which potencies are most used in everyday practice?*

A: That depends on the nature of the illness and the constitution of the patient. The decision is very individual, whether a 30C, 200C, 1M, 10M or an LM is used.

Q: *When I buy a homœopathic remedy in a pharmacy I have to take five globules at least three times daily before the symptoms improve. I have just been to a homœopath. I merely got a little packet of five globules to take once. My next appointment is a month away. Can this remedy possibly work?*

A: The remedy you have received from your homœopath is presumably in high potency, i.e., it is active for longer, often for months, and acts on a deeper level than those over-the-counter remedies.

Q: *In a lecture I heard that a constitutional remedy was for life, i.e. always the same remedy would be prescribed. I find it difficult to imagine, that it's that simple. People change too, shouldn't the remedy?*

A: You are quite right. It is seldom the case that a single remedy is the answer. Particularly in "complex" illnesses several remedies are required at greater intervals. And it is rare that a person requires the same remedy all their life, from childhood to adulthood.

Q: *My homœopath never tells me what homœopathic remedy he has prescribed. Is there a reason for this?*

A: Yes, namely for the reason that you can allow the remedy to work without bias or prejudice. In practice it has been shown that patients who know their remedy and look it up in the lay literature, are often prejudiced and can no longer judge their reactions with true objectivity. But there is no reason not to mention the name of the remedy at a later date.

Q: *I am 72 years old and have been subjected to numerous operations, and suffer from several ailments. Now I feel that I want to try a different approach as far as my health is concerned. Is there any point at my age? Can homœopathy help me despite my many operations and earlier treatment?*

A: Age does not matter in homœopathy. With the correct homœopathic treatment even a weakened Vital Force can be strengthened. Obviously, this will require some time and patience. Organic changes cannot be reversed. But it has been shown that a person, strengthened internally and more balanced through homœopathy, can better come to terms with their complaints. Their quality of life is enhanced, and further illnesses can be prevented.

Q: *I am pregnant and want to avoid any medication so as not to injure my unborn child. What is the situation on side-effects with homœopathic remedies?*

A: You can rest assured. Taken in the correct dosage, homœopathic remedies are quite harmless. On this subject we point you to Chapter: Homœopathy During Pregnancy.

Q: *From what age can one be treated homœo-pathically?*

A: Treatment is already possible during birth. Homœo-pathically-trained midwives are having great success with it. They give the newborn a remedy immediately after the birth, where necessary.

Q: *Recently I was searching the Internet for infor-mation on homœopathy. It was very overwhelming. I found hundreds of different addresses.*

A: You can save yourself this effort. At www.groma.ch you will find a worldwide collection of the most important links on Classical Homœopathy. You may also like to try www.homeopathhome.com or www.homeopath.co.uk.

Bibliography

- Blackie, Margery Dr, *Classical Homœopathy* (1986) Beaconsfield: Beaconsfield Publishers Ltd
- Blackie, Margery Dr, *The Patient Not The Cure* (1976) London: MacDonald & Jane's
- Castro, Miranda, *The Complete Homœopathy Handbook* (1990) London: Macmillan
- Curtis, Susan, *A Handbook of Homœopathic Alternatives to Immunisation* (1996) London: Winter Press
- Gunn, Trevor, *Mass Immunisation. A Point in Question* (1992) Kendal: Cutting Edge Publications
- Hahnemann, Samuel, *Organon of medicine,* 6th Edition, Delhi: B. Jain Publishers
- Kent, JT, *Lectures on Homœopathic Philosophy,* Delhi: B. Jain Publishers
- Köhler, Gerhard, *The Handbook of Homœopathy,* Delhi: B. Jain Publishers
- Vithoulkas, George, *The Science of Homœopathy*
- Vithoulkas, George, *Homœopathy – Medicine of the New Man* (1985) London: Thorsons
- Vithoulkas, George, *A New Model for Health and Disease* (1991) Berkley: North Atlantic Books

Addresses

Helios Homœopathic Pharmacy
89-97 Camden Road
Tunbridge Wells
Kent TN1 2QR
Tel. 01892-537254/536393 (24 hrs)
http://www.helios.co.uk

Nelsons Homœopathic Pharmacy
73 Duke Street
Grosvenor Square
London W1M 6BY
Tel. 020-7495-2404

Book distribution, further information on obtaining
first aid kits and courses, contact:

Hans G Schrauder BSc LCH MHMA MGCP
The Homœopathic Clinic
82 Amberwood Rise
New Malden KT3 5JQ
Tel. 020-8942-2668
Email: the.homoeopath@virgin.net

or at

The Eden Medical Centre
63a Kings Road
London SW3 4NT
Tel. 020-7881-5800
Email: hs@edenmedicalcentre.com